HOW TO STAY HEALTHY IN A WORLD DESIGNED TO MAKE US FAT AND LAZY

By
LORIE EBER

By Lorie Eber, JD, Mayo Clinic Certified Wellness Coach, NASM Certified Personal Trainer

Text copyright © 2015 by Lorie Eber

All rights reserved

ISBN-10: 1508608350

ISBN-13: 9781508608356

TABLE OF CONTENTS

Table of Contents iii
Dedication v
Introduction vii

Guiding Strategies

The Three Causes of Obesity: SOS 3
How Did We Get Fat and Lazy? 7
Your Body Houses Your Soul: Get a Clue 9
The Three Counterintuitive Secrets to Staying Healthy 11
The Five Secrets to Lifestyle Change 15
A Month's Worth of Daily Health Tips 19

Eat Less Garbage

My Journey to Vegetarianism and Back 23
The Colon Cleanse Has Become the New Penance 27
Leave Dr. Oz in the Land of Oz 29
So You Think Gourmet Food Is Healthy? 31
Don't Go Through Another Molting Season 33
Six Diet and Nutrition Myths Debunked 39

Why We Keep Doing Something with a
95 Percent Failure Rate 43

Mid-February Might Be a Good Time for
That New Year's Resolution. 47

Lose That Depression Mentality to Stay Healthy 49

Get That Body Moving

Confessions of a Fitness Fanatic. 53

A Surefire Way to Rev Up Your Metabolism 55

My Top Ten Peeves at the Gym 59

Exer-Snacks: The Best Way to Get Your
Body Moving 63

The Downside of Being Fit and Lean 67

Take Your Stress Down a Notch

Can a Type A Learn to Meditate?. 73

Three Tips for Stressed-Out Professionals 77

How to Maintain Your Sanity during the Holidays 81

Are You Too Busy to Go to the Restroom? 83

Slow Down: Get Your Stress Down to a
Reasonable Level 85

Lorie Eber's Bio 89

DEDICATION

This book is dedicated to my wonderful husband, Wes, who brings joy to my life!

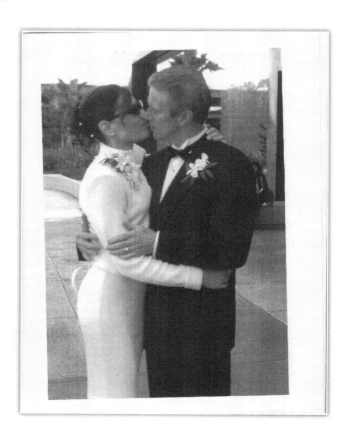

INTRODUCTION

In the old days, when portion sizes were appropriate and our ancestors were accustomed to walking as a regular means of transportation, it was relatively easy to maintain the weight your body was intended to carry. Today, staying healthy often feels like a Sisyphean task because we now live in a cultural environment conducive to excessive eating and sitting. While bucking the tide can make you feel like a salmon swimming upstream, it is perfectly doable with a little strategizing and planning.

This book will give you all the tools you need to enjoy good health. I'll help you cut though all the noise and contradictory advice and give you simple techniques that will help you avoid the ubiquitous signals that cause us to eat more than our body needs and to remain deskbound. It's not complicated. I'll give you all the skills you need to successfully change your habits. You probably won't go from a couch potato to working out four to five hours a day and having a body like Jillian Michaels, but with time and a little patience, you can certainly get back to a healthy BMI.

GUIDING STRATEGIES

We'd all like to be in shape, but we need some reasonable principles to consistently follow to resist the lure of this week's Dr. Oz remedy. Here are some simple rules that will help keep you on the straight and narrow.

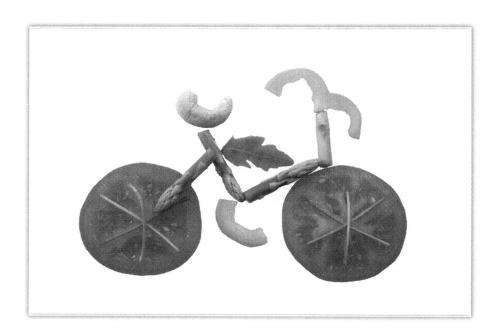

THE THREE CAUSES OF OBESITY: SOS

We're in the midst of an obesity epidemic, which is leading to chronic diseases like type 2 diabetes at never-before-seen rates. Have you ever wondered why this is happening? I've boiled it down to three simple causes, synopsized with the apropos acronym SOS.

1. **Seats**

We're constantly implored to "take a seat." Most of us sit all day at our desks, during interminable meetings, and while commuting, and then cap off the day reclining on the couch while gorging on mindless entertainment. We now know that seats are hazardous to our health. They should come with a cigarette-like warning that says, "Prolonged sitting leads to high blood pressure, obesity, diabetes, heart disease, depression, and even death." Research supports those dire predictions. A well-documented study of twelve thousand Australians concluded that those who watched TV for six hours per day shortened their lifespans by 4.8 years. While you might not be a telly addict of that order, a sedentary occupation will yield the same result. Your body doesn't know if you're sitting for work or pleasure. You can't fight biology. Our bodies yearn to emulate the Energizer Bunny. Instead of always plunking ourselves down in a comfy chair, our default position should be standing up and moving. Perhaps cheapo Ryanair should tack on an upcharge for the health benefits conferred by its vertical seats.

2. **Outsourcing**

Are you old enough to remember when meals were made from scratch in our own kitchens? These days, home-cooked meals have been relegated to a special occasion aberration. Sometimes I wonder why homebuilders bother installing kitchen ovens. Today we outsource our food preparation. We scarf down food with one hand on the wheel or eat a day's worth of calories at lunch by inhaling a huge salad swimming in tasty ranch dressing. We've decided we don't have time to cook anymore. Most of us consider what we put into our bodies so inconsequential that we shove it in while working at our desks or binge-watching Netflix. Eating out has become a time-saving convenience and a way for foodies to entertain themselves. It's not only our wallets that suffer from eating out. Our bellies tell the tale since the average restaurant diner consumes two hundred more calories than someone who eats a meal at home.

The culprits are a caloric trifecta of gobs of flavor-enhancing butter, indulging in the oft-made suggestion of "calamari for the table," and the sheeple behavior of ordering dessert just because your dining companions say the crème brûlée is "to die for." Since the likelihood of returning to the days of June Cleaver is nil, here are two practical ideas. Shop for nourishing food on the weekend so you can throw a meal together in under five minutes, and stash wholesome snacks in your office. If money is no object, buy prepared foods from upscale grocers like Whole Foods or order home delivery from a healthy gourmet purveyor. You do remember how to use the microwave, don't you?

3. **Science Projects**

We used to eat real food that came from animals and from the soil. Now we eat science projects concocted in Nestle, General Mills, PepsiCo, and ConAgra plants. Extensive research goes into fabricating just the right combinations of tastes that will light up the pleasure centers in our brains in ways that are eerily similar to snorting cocaine. Then, they seal the deal by constantly hawking these chemical compounds in print, television, and social media. You shouldn't need linguistics training to be able to understand an ingredient label. Nor should a chemistry degree be a prerequisite to decipher the long list of mystery additives. Mike Pollan's Food Rule #19 is a good rule of thumb: "If it came from a plant, eat it; if it was made in a plant, don't."

HOW DID WE GET FAT AND LAZY?

Why do two-thirds of American adults now shop for XXL sizes and huff and puff on the rare occasions they are forced to walk more than fifty feet?

Is it due to "fat" genes? Lack of information about nutrition or exercise regimens? The purportedly high cost of fresh fruits and vegetables? A conspiracy by the processed food industry? That evil Ronald McDonald and his brethren? Or is an epidemic of immediate gratification sweeping the country?

My answer: none of the above. The villain? Our modern lifestyle and work habits practically guarantee that most of us will resemble Humpy-Dumpty rather than the buffed athlete with the perfect physique who adorns the Wheaties box.

It's easy to see how we develop the habit of overeating. Inexpensive, high-calorie food is available 24-7 everywhere. Just cruise through the drive-thru, walk through the office kitchen, or put your coins in the vending machine. Want a sit-down meal? You won't do any better. Order a meal in any restaurant from fast casual to pricey gourmet, and your server will deliver a football player–size hunk of protein and enough starch to feed an impoverished nation. What you won't get is more than three pieces of plant material.

Not moving our bodies has become as natural as incessantly checking our smartphones. I grew up accustomed to using my legs for transportation and sprinting whenever a cabbie tried to make me into a flattened cartoon character. But New York City is an aberration. Most locales cater only to four-wheeled vehicles. Sidewalks have become unreliable. Without warning, they come to a screeching halt, and you're forced into the street. Hoofing it through a mall parking lot instead of parking directly in front of your favorite store is tantamount to a death wish.

Most of us are desk jockeys. We obediently sit and stare at a computer screen, entranced, for eight hours or more. Those motion-sensor lights are so annoying when they decide there's no sign of human life in your office and leave you in the dark. Don't know about you, but I feel slightly foolish waving my arms to prove I'm still breathing.

Some of us are even reluctant to drink water because it might precipitate a bathroom break. We can't fit that into our busy schedules. Leaving our electronic post for even a few minutes is tantamount to shirking our job responsibilities.

The ubiquitous drive-thru represents the epitome of our sedentary, multitasking lives. It provides an unparalleled opportunity to remain completely immobile while unconsciously devouring junk food, checking our e-mail, and trying to drive without hitting anything large enough to put a big dent in our SUV.

But is this any way to live? Aren't we going to pay a price for our self-neglect at some point? You bet. We already are. The annual medical cost of obesity, according to the Centers for Disease Control and Prevention, is a whopping $147 billion.

It's not that we're not trying to lose weight. After all, someone is fueling the $40 billion weight-loss industry. The problem is that the "quick fix" doesn't change lifestyles. It only prolongs the agony by starting an endless cycle of shedding and reacquiring the same pounds.

The key? Be a realist. Start changing your lifestyle by setting small, achievable goals. Create accountability. Celebrate small victories. Focus on the positive—getting healthier. Avoid the scale. And most important: Don't even think about making any change that you can't sustain for the rest of your life!

YOUR BODY HOUSES YOUR SOUL: GET A CLUE

Most of us cycle through the pattern of overeating, dieting, and then rebelling against our self-imposed list of forbidden foods. Others are bound and determined to sweat off the excess baggage by plunking down a hefty sum for a long-term gym membership. For added motivation, why not sign up for a prepaid package of personal training sessions? The usual result — when the buffed specimen asks them to re-up, they disappear from the health club, never to be seen again, until they repeat the cycle.

The more frugal among us buys a treadmill or exercise bike and vows to use it every evening after work. Almost as soon as it's set up, it becomes apparent that there are so many other things to do in the evening, all of which seem like more fun than working out on a machine while your brain screams, "I don't want to do this!" Before long, the home gym gathers dust and acts as a clothes drop.

Then there's the lure of the magic pill. The placebo effect of downing Dr. Oz–endorsed miracle fat melters may trick your brain for a while, but then you wise up and stop wasting your hard-earned cash. Sadly, the health-and-fitness industry is only too happy to grab for our wallets as we cycle through fitness trends over and over, like serial daters.

The stark fact is that two-thirds of the population is now overweight or obese. We're taxing our bodies every day with excess weight that it's not equipped to handle, ingesting way more calories than we need, and making very little attempt to make use of that fuel by moving our bodies.

We all understand the importance of taking care of our bodies. And, at times, we do focus on eating a healthy diet and on getting moving. But, most often, we choose to make our health a low priority. We tell ourselves that we're just too busy to pay attention to what we eat or to make time to work out. Mind you, we intend to start—real soon.

If we've been blessed with good genetics, our bodies can put up with years of neglect and abuse before signaling the point of no return. Suddenly, it seems, our body is falling apart. The breakdown may take the form of a chronic disease like diabetes or inflict unrelenting back or joint pain. Yet even this loud wake-up call frequently elicits only a short-lived response. Most often, we decide to succumb to the quick fix—drugs or surgery.

Let me suggest a way out of this start-stop conundrum. How about if we get literal? As Jim Rohn, the well-known entrepreneur and motivational speaker, put it, "Take care of your body. It's the only place you have to live." How about if we started treating our bodies at least as well as our homes?

You maintain your home, don't you? You pick up all the kids' toys. Take out the trash. Vacuum up the dirt the dog dragged in. Run the dishwasher after dinner. You even do the gross stuff, like cleaning the bathroom. Bottom line: somehow you find the time and money to devote to the upkeep of your abode.

Doesn't your body, the precious vehicle that houses your soul and has amazing, life-sustaining automatic functions, deserve at least comparable devotion? Try on the idea. It just might give you the motivation to put health maintenance on the front burner.

THE THREE COUNTERINTUITIVE SECRETS TO STAYING HEALTHY

Be a little indulgent. Be a little wimpy. Be a little imperfect. I'm suggesting that we resist the temptation to set ridiculously high standards for ourselves when we periodically get disgusted with ourselves. Instead, we should focus on healthy behaviors.

This may sound counterintuitive, but it's the only effective coping mechanism in a culture that conspires to make us fat, lazy, and stressed out. Unfortunately, drive-thrus are here to stay, another over-the-top exercise regime will replace CrossFit when it becomes passé, and the demands of your 24-7 workplace are not going to ease up so that you can have a lovely, balanced life. This is our reality, and we need to learn to live in it.

We all know the ingredients of a healthy, happy life: managing stress, eating healthy foods, and keeping our bodies moving. Yet many of us never manage to get these under control. Instead, we ricochet between healthy and unhealthy phases. We go on diets. We hire personal trainers. We say "om." We're doing great…for a while. But then, we lose our resolve. We go to Carl's Jr. and order a half-pound Western Bacon Thickburger with fries. We sit on the couch and eat our way through a bag of Lay's Cheddar Bacon Mac & Cheese chips. We put on our makeup and check our phones while on the way to work and cause a fender bender.

Why can't we stay on the straight and narrow? Why do we keep vacillating between "being good" and acting like a hedonist? As ironic as it may seem, the problem is that we try to be "too good." We set the bar too high, fail, get discouraged, and give up.

Let's say you convince yourself that sugar is evil and decide to cut out all desserts. You may succeed in abiding by this draconian rule for a week or two, but when your birthday rolls around and you're presented with a homemade chocolate fudge cake, you indulge. The first piece tastes like nirvana. Before you know it, you've wolfed down a second piece. You feel guilty, but you give yourself a "birthday exception" and fully intend to resume your saintly ways. Instead, you slide down the slippery slope. The first time you have a rough day at work, you find yourself in bed binging on Ben & Jerry's while overindulging in episodes of *Orange Is the New Black*.

Stop Trying to Be a Mother Teresa

1. **Be a little indulgent.** Don't put any food on the "forbidden" list. It will call your name. Even if you splurge on a nutritionally bankrupt yet oh-so-tempting deep-fried treat at the county fair, indulging once in a while isn't not going to give you thunder thighs or add two inches to your waist.

2. **Be a little wimpy.** Unless you're already in great shape, super-strenuous workouts like CrossFit are not for you. And many personal trainers are on a mission to give you the toughest, never-to-be-repeated workout of your life. The predictable result: injury or burnout. You don't need to be that macho; be a little wimpy instead. The key is to discover some fun, or at least tolerable, ways to get your body moving that you won't come to dread.

3. Be a little imperfect. Much of our stress is caused by a drive to be perfect — as a parent, as an employee, as a boss. Abandon that unattainable goal. You can't be all things to all people 24-7 and also give yourself the time and attention you need to recharge and stay healthy. Be content with being slightly less than perfect.

THE FIVE SECRETS TO LIFESTYLE CHANGE

I'm a trained wellness coach and certified personal trainer, and I have helped many clients make permanent lifestyle changes. It's not an easy thing to do. Look around. There's no escaping the fact that our environment is sedentary and supersized. Fast-food drive-thrus are ubiquitous and most of us are tethered to our desks. This is our reality, and we need to learn to find a way live in the real world, rather than grasping at the latest, greatest miracle weight-loss solution. McDonald's is not going out of business any time soon. Nor are we about to return to our ancestral hunter-gatherer ways.

Staying healthy in this setting can seem like an insurmountable hurdle—one that requires 24-7 diligence. Sometimes you'll feel like you're in a rip current. While this is a formidable challenge, it is doable, and it trumps feeling lousy, living on meds, and eventually dealing with chronic illness.

I have distilled the five secrets that hold the key to making lasting lifestyle changes:

#1: **Emulate the tortoise, not the hare.** Most people who get fed up with themselves make shortsighted moves like going on diets or depleting their bank accounts for gym memberships.

Chances are they've tried both before, were rewarded with short-term gains, and eventually returned to the habits that got them into trouble in the first place. Get off the weight roller coaster. Don't panic, and try to turn yourself into a kale-eating gym rat overnight. Try small, gradual adjustments that don't send your body into shock and leave you feeling deprived and exhausted.

#2: Be an Underachiever. Every time you decide on a lifestyle tweak, ask yourself, "Is this something that I can do for the rest of my life?" If the answer is anything other than a resounding yes, don't go there. If beef is "what's for dinner" in your world, don't resolve to go cold turkey and never eat red meat again. You're setting yourself up for failure. I promise you that as soon as your fire up your backyard BBQ and get a whiff of that cheeseburger, it will scream, "Eat me! Eat me!" and you will succumb. A more practical goal would be to cut back your beef consumption from seven to five times a week. Be realistic, not extreme.

#3: Take "exer-snacks." Change your attitude about exercise. My parents never made a concerted effort to exercise, yet they were in good shape. Broaden your horizons. Look for excuses to move your body throughout the day. Latch onto any pretext, no matter how flimsy, to get up and move. Consider a stand-up desk. Host walking meetings. Pace up and down during conference calls. Take the stairs. Little things add up on the exercise front. Get away from the mind-set that "working out" means going the gym for ninety minutes. Find things you actually like to do. It might be line dancing or digging in the dirt. You don't have to kill yourself to stay in shape.

#4: View weight loss as a "happy by-product." Don't make your bathroom scale the barometer of your self-worth. The weight will come off, but to banish it for good, you have to ride the local train, not the supersonic jet. You didn't gain twenty-five pounds in three weeks, and you can't safely lose it in that time frame. Be patient and step away from the scale. Otherwise, you'll quickly get discouraged and descend into the black hole.

#5: Be a little bad. There's no need to join the nunnery or a monastery to be healthy. Give yourself permission to be a little bad. Food is one of the most enjoyable aspects of life. If your favorite treat is Ben & Jerry's Chubby Hubby, don't ever make it verboten. Allow yourself to enjoy it—just find your own personal moderation solution.

Keep these five rules in mind, and you can change your life for good!

A MONTH'S WORTH OF DAILY HEALTH TIPS

1. Eat at home and save two hundred calories per day.
2. Multitasking leads to eating amnesia.
3. Think about foods to add to your diet rather than making a list of forbidden foods.
4. Store the healthy foods front and center in your fridge.
5. The average person underestimates calorie consumption by more than 20 percent.
6. When eating out, ask to sub the starch for more vegetables.
7. If you snack after dinner, journal how you feel to identify the trigger and find something healthier to fill the need.
8. Eat breakfast like a king, lunch like a prince, and dinner like a pauper.
9. Download restaurant menus before you leave home and make a healthy selection.
10. Split a salad and an entrée when dining out.
11. Eat with healthy people, and mimic their choices.
12. Get adequate sleep so that your hunger hormones are reset.

13. Drink water throughout the day so you don't mistake thirst for hunger.
14. Avoid the middle aisles at the grocery stores.
15. Institute a one-day-a-week cheat day to "be a little bad."
16. Create accountability by telling everyone you know that you have resolved to eat healthier.
17. Do three ten-minute exer-snacks to sneak in your exercise.
18. Get a stand-up desk so you don't sit for extended periods and slow blood flow.
19. Get a fitness tracker to monitor your steps.
20. Think of exercising as moving your body, not as forcing yourself to go to the gym.
21. Take the stairs instead of the elevator.
22. Add resistance training to your routine, and you can eat more.
23. Consider getting dog that you'll have to walk twice a day.
24. Start a diet from a place of self-love and acceptance.
25. Set goals that are so specific that you can't wiggle out of them.
26. Forgive yourself as you would a loved one when you don't meet one of your goals.
27. Incorporate some gratitude into your life each day.
28. Do something kind for someone else to lift your spirits.
29. Record your workouts in your smartphone like any other appointments.
30. Plan to eat well, and it will happen.

EAT LESS GARBAGE

Most of us who are overweight are just eating more food than our bodies need. Remember that dessert you ate last evening because it looked too good to pass up and those chips you munched on when you wanted something crunchy? Guess what? Those extra calories didn't dissipate into thin air. They ended up on your belly, hips, or thighs.

We also tend to eat science projects rather than real food. Chemical concoctions are packed with calories, whereas vegetables, fruits, and lean protein are not. An easy way to eat better is to choose mostly plants, which allows you the visual of a full plate without the temptation of overeating.

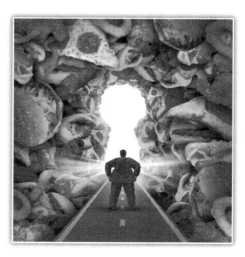

MY JOURNEY TO VEGETARIANISM AND BACK

When I was thirteen years old, I made a rash decision to swear off eating all animals. Forever. My epiphany was grounded in the idealistic notion that my selfish need for protein was a wholly insufficient reason to decapitate a chicken. Mind you, I grew up in New York City and had never even seen a chicken, except perhaps at the Children's Zoo in Central Park. My juvenile empathy did not extend to my mother, who was then burdened with making two separate dinners every evening so that the rest of the family could continue to eat normally.

In retrospect, my true motivator may have been run-of-the-mill adolescent rebellion. After all, my health-conscious mother had sent me off to school every day with an untradeable healthy sandwich on rock-hard Pepperidge Farm bread and two carrot sticks. Why wasn't I allowed to enjoy the wonderfully squishy Wonder Bread all my friends loved? My distaste for meat may have been prompted by my mother's paranoia of undercooking it, which resulted in plates of overcooked, gray-colored flesh with a leather-shoe consistency. Can you say "yummy?"

Mom also tried in vain to ration the sweet treats every kid craves. Her strategy was to padlock the goodies away in the far reaches of the cabinet above the refrigerator. She should have known better than to try to get between kids and their favorite cookies. We evaded her well-intentioned efforts by shimmying our little hands through the miniscule opening and grabbing whatever was reachable. Skinned hands were a small price to pay to feed our insatiable sweet tooths.

For the next fourteen years, no chicken, cow, or pig parts touched my lips. My diet consisted mainly of starches, high-fat dairy, and desserts. I decided vegetables were boring and ate few of them. Essentially, I was on the very junk-food diet my mother had worked so valiantly to have me avoid. I remained blissfully unaware that my restrictive diet scored near zero on the health barometer.

Except for some leftover hippies, I was an oddity as a noncarnivore in the seventies and eighties. Many people treated me as if I was doing something quite admirable, thinking it involved a herculean dose of self-restraint. Mistakenly assuming I subsisted on raw vegetables and tasteless tofu, they expressed admiration for my purported willpower.

Once I started practicing law, I moved to Chicago and was taken aback to discover that I was living in the meat eater's capital of the country. Natives couldn't fathom getting through breakfast without a slab of crisp bacon or a few links of Polish sausage. Things got uncomfortable when I was required to dine with law-firm clients, who looked askance as I tried to make a meal out of cottage cheese and a double serving of creamed spinach. I often wondered if they were asking themselves, "Do I really want to entrust my legal problems to this nonmeat-eating wacko?"

Meanwhile, I continued to get my daily fill of Dr. Peppers, Cokes, Snickers bars, Ding Dongs, and Hostess cupcakes with squiggles on top. I made weekly forays to my local Woolworth counter to scarf down a gooey banana split. A large bowl of generously buttered popcorn was my go-to dinner.

That was my version of a vegetarian diet. I've known many a nonmeat-eater who follows a very similar diet regimen. After all, it's the perfect excuse to indulge in tasty but nutritionally bankrupt fare. No animal ever died in the name of delectable pumpkin cheesecake, flourless chocolate cake, or crème brûlée. Far from depriving myself, I now realize that I was actually indulging in chemically ladened processed garbage. So much for being holier than thou.

One day, as impulsively as I'd decided to banish animals from my diet, I reversed course and made a snap decision to revert to a normal diet. I'd gotten to the point where I realized I really didn't care that much about the stupid chickens. Off with their heads! By this time, it had also dawned on me that my nonmeat-eating habits were probably not doing my body a world of good.

Once having made the call to rejoin the American way of life, I worried that when animal flesh hit my gut, my body would imitate Linda Blair in *The Exorcist*. I tested the waters with Chinese food, assured that the chicken serving would be garnish sized. Much to my relief, I discovered that my body had not misplaced its carnivore digestive juices despite years of disuse.

Since seeing the error of my ways, I have gradually gravitated to a healthy Mediterranean diet, which allows for a reasonable and enjoyable life. I eat mostly vegetables and fruit, some complex carbs, and small amounts of fish and chicken. Ironically, I am much closer to being a true vegetarian today than I ever was when I declared myself one as a naïve teenager.

THE COLON CLEANSE HAS BECOME THE NEW PENANCE

Colon cleanses are all the rage. Many people have convinced themselves that they need to rid their bodies of the "lethal toxins" which have built up, like so much drain-clogging gunk, due to their poor lifestyle choices. We're talking months of McD's drive-thrus, colossal-sized Claim Jumper dinners, Cronut breakfasts, and midnight binges with Benny & Jerry.

There are a variety of body-cleansing versions of Drano available — juice concoctions, pills containing "all-natural herbs," enemas, or laxatives, singly or in combination. I've often wondered why the GI docs don't take advantage of this trend and tell their patients that colonoscopy prep is just a colon cleanse. They might get more takers.

Detoxing isn't pleasant, but that's the whole point. It involves starving yourself, drinking noxious fluids, enduring GI cramps, and visiting the bathroom more often than someone with food poisoning. But that's all fine because you feel you deserve it. After all, you know you've abused your body. Bring on the warranted punishment! As an added benefit, you'll probably lose a few pounds due to calorie deprivation. It might just be the jumpstart you need to finally start losing those extra ten pounds. Or has it gone up to twenty? So, what's not to like?

This self-inflicted punishment strikes me as the bodily equivalent of going to the Catholic priest, copping to your misdeeds, performing the prescribed penance, having your sins washed away, and starting anew. It's like Larry Hagman getting a new liver after destroying his first one or Jimmy Carter confessing that he'd lusted in his heart for women other than Rosalynn. In some twisted way, you enjoy the self-punishment of the cleanse. You get to start over, tabula rasa.

The only problem is that this ablution, like the vaginal douche, is based on a faulty premise. It presumes that the human body is incapable of processing food and ridding itself of the unabsorbed by-products. Since many of us lack a basic understanding of our own bodily functions and imagine that our insides look like a greasy community BBQ grill, we fall prey to the delusion that we need to follow a prescribed regimen to remove the aftermath of too many servings of burgers and fries. In fact, the body has amazingly efficient self-cleaning organs, the liver and kidneys, which work miraculously well to process what we eat and to remove the waste products.

The truth is that a colon cleanse is unnecessary at best and may even put your health at risk. A recent examination of twenty studies on the topic by Georgetown University researchers found "absolutely no evidence that colon cleansing helps. Instead, we found that it can be harmful." Potential dangers include cramping, bloating, vomiting, electrolyte imbalance, renal failure, and even death.

We need to fashion a better way to beat ourselves up after we overindulge. How about something like traffic school—perhaps a pricey, mandatory, day-long course in human physiology? What are your suggestions for public self-flagellation?

LEAVE DR. OZ IN THE LAND OF OZ

My healthy-living message is simple: eat nutritious food in reasonable amounts, move your body more, and manage your stress. It's not rocket science. You don't need to be a registered dietician to know that a salmon and broccoli dinner is a better choice than a Carl's Jr. Double Western Double Cheeseburger with large fries. Of course, it's seductively easy to succumb to the pleasures of high-fat, super-caloric foods. While eating comfort food may provide immediate gratification and serve as a reward after a stressful day, the inevitable outcome is that your body starts to resemble an In-N-Out Double-Double. What do you do then? You look for a quick fix, of course. And you want to take off the added baggage immediately, if not sooner. So, why go through the agony of making lifestyle changes when you can just down a pill? It's the American way.

Who's the go-to guy for the quick fix? How about a well-respected cardiac surgeon, a professor of surgery at Columbia University, and the esteemed director of the Cardiovascular Institute and Complementary Medicine Program at New York Presbyterian Hospital? If these credentials don't impress you, he's also a prolific writer, author of seven *New York Times* best sellers, and *Forbes* Most Influential Celebrity of 2010–11. Thanks to Oprah, he graces the airways daily.

Unless you've been holed up in an ashram for the last decade, you know that I'm referring to none other than Dr. Oz. His imprimatur is so powerful that any fat-burning pill he mentions on his daily television show flies off the shelves immediately. Currently, the quick-weight-loss guru is trumpeting garcinia cambogia, a small fruit also known as a tamarind, as "the most exciting breakthrough in weight loss to date." Wait a minute. In the past, he's recommended raspberry ketones, green coffee bean extract, African mango, red palm oil, acai berry extract, saffron extract, and 7-Keto DHEA as fat-incinerating breakthroughs. With all these miracles under his belt, Dr. Oz must be a shoo-in for canonization.

The fact that Dr. Oz's audience continues to trek to GNC, clutching hope in the form of a scrawled note with the name of the latest Oz-recommended pill, is a testament to how difficult it is to change our habits. Convenient, inexpensive fast food in supersize portions is everywhere. Workplace kitchens seem to spawn an endless supply of donuts, cookies, chocolates, and leftover cake. Receptions and fatty hors d'oeuvres go hand in hand. Restaurant entrées serve three, and then the waiter asks, "Have you saved room for dessert?" Is it any wonder we overindulge?

Unfortunately, no matter how many overnight-weight-loss solutions Dr. Oz trumpets, none actually work. The only way to avoid joining the ranks of the 69.2 percent of adults in the United States that are overweight or obese is to accept the calories in, calories out equation as your reality. Habit change is a step-by-step process that takes time and patience. The twenty to thirty extra pounds did not appear overnight and will not melt like spring snow, no matter how many pills you take. If you shed it quickly, your resolve will eventually weaken, and the extra pounds will find you again. My advice: take it slow — be a tortoise, not a hare.

SO YOU THINK GOURMET FOOD IS HEALTHY?

My boomer and Gen Y friends are obsessed with food. They live and breathe gourmet restaurants and celebrity chefs. To them, gastronomical creations are "to die for!" Many of them subscribe to the nutrition myth that gourmet food is healthy food.

They avoid the drive-thru, realizing that fried food, mega doses of salt, and supersize meals do not lead to stellar yearly checkups. They also wouldn't be caught dead in TGI Fridays or the Cheesecake Factory. Nutritionally speaking, that's a good thing. A whopping 96 percent of the entrées served at those eateries exceed the recommendations for fat and sodium set by USDA. Maybe that's because the portions are two to eight times the recommended serving sizes.

My food-aficionado friends consider themselves a cut above the riffraff as they eagerly seek out the grand opening of Wolfgang Puck's or Gordon Ramsey's latest culinary adventure to indulge in the delectable tasting menu. For the food devotee, the pièce de résistance is dining at Per Se on a special occasion. Order from Thomas Keller's tasting menu, and you will delight in Tsar Imperial Caviar, Elevanges Perigord Foie Gras, Snake River Farms Calotte De Boeuf, and Champlain Valley's Triple Cream, to name just a few. While indulging in this gastronomic feast, it's easy to overlook the fact that this taste-bud extravaganza set you back 2,320 calories. To put this in perspective, a Big Mac, an order of large fries, and a thirty-two-ounce regular Coke weighs in at a mere 1,360 calories.

Admittedly, treating yourself to a ten-course meal is not an everyday occurrence. Many of us, including myself, frequent the upscale restaurants where dining is treated as an event on par with attending a Broadway show or an art gallery opening. The diners speak "Gourmandese" when they order: "I think I'll do the Colorado Buffalo Carpaccio tonight." The menu descriptions are so obtuse, you'd have to Google the ingredients to make an intelligent selection, but it's more fun to just be surprised. When dining with a group of friends, an order of fried calamari is the table centerpiece. Of course, you must try a few scrumptious desserts. Rumor has it that so long as you share, these sweets have almost no calories.

I hate to admit it, but gourmet restaurant offerings are not particularly healthy either. Replacing the description "deep fried" with the chichi terms "fritto misto," crispy skin," or "panko crusted" does not remove the oil. Crème fraiche, beurre blanc, and béchamel sauces may sound fancy, but they're still fat pills. The ugly truth is that all restaurant food is loaded with butter and salt. That's why it tastes so good.

Almost makes you want to stay home and cook, doesn't it? But then what would we do for entertainment?

DON'T GO THROUGH ANOTHER MOLTING SEASON

For many of the two-thirds of Americans who are overweight or obese, maintaining a healthy weight is a lifelong battle somewhat akin to molting. Although they are able to muster the willpower to deprive themselves and lose excess baggage, they simply can't maintain their hard-earned weight loss. They may be overlooking the three strategies that are critical to maintaining a healthy weight.

The one hundred million Americans who are dieting at any given time often have multiple wardrobes to accommodate their seesaw girth. When they can no longer zip up their "fat jeans," it's time to shed again. While calorie-restrictive regimens and other quick-weight-loss schemes often work, they are only a temporary reprieve from the fat suit, which almost always reappears, oftentimes in a larger size.

This never-ending quest to lose weight supports a $20 billion industry. Hope springs eternal despite repeated failures. We want to believe that somehow, someday, we will find a way to recapture our high-school physique.

There are more weight-loss schemes than cockroaches in New York City apartments. Nutrisystem will sell you prepackaged meals so you don't have figure out what to put in your mouth. A new diet seems to pop up every day. The latest darlings are the fast diet, the paleo diet, the cabbage soup diet, and the master cleanse. So many people have jumped on the gluten-free bandwagon that it has exploded into a $4.4 billion per year industry, despite overwhelming evidence that shunning wheat products does not promote weight loss. Shop at GNC or Whole Foods, and you'll find an astounding array of pills that supposedly melt away fat. Unfortunately, the only long-lasting effect of any of these strategies is a lighter bank account.

While calories in, calories out is the undeniable metric, people who want to banish excess pounds often inadvertently undermine their valiant efforts by overlooking the three indispensable elements that hold the key to ending the yo-yo dieting syndrome.

Here's what you need to do: 1. eat breakfast every day, 2. get adequate shut-eye, and 3. make exercise a part of everyday life.

Thirty-one million Americans skip breakfast every day. Some say they aren't hungry in the morning, while others are just too busy to give their body the fuel it needs to get going. But don't fool yourself. This is not a way to "save calories." On the contrary. That donut in the office kitchen will pop into your mouth, or you'll opt for the greasy burger place for lunch and supersize it.

More than a dozen studies document the association between eating a healthy breakfast and weight control. Breaking the fast in the morning yields other benefits too, including healthier food choices throughout the day and an improved ability to think straight and concentrate.

Do you try to pack more into your busy day by trying to scrape by on four hours of sleep? Think again. Lack of sleep and being overweight are inextricably linked. Scientists have identified a brain chemical, adenosine, responsible for promoting sleepiness. Without sufficient rest, this substance does not fully flush out of our system, and we still feel sluggish. When our bodies are sleep deprived, we crave high-calorie, high-fat foods. In a recent study, bleary-eyed subjects consumed six hundred more calories per day than those who had slept eight hours.

The third critical component that will cause you to smile when you hop off the scale is consistent exercise. Of the ten thousand people being tracked by the National Weight Control Registry, 90 percent exercise for an hour every day. Many experts believe that regular exercise may be more critical to preventing the excess weight from creeping back on than to losing the weight in the first place. And you don't have to kill yourself. Walking at a brisk pace is effective.

Give these three weight-maintenance strategies a try. You'll only need one wardrobe, and you'll never have to go through another molting season.

Follow These Simple Strategies to Lose Weight for Good

When we get disgusted with our weight, we go on a diet because usually it results in rapid weight loss, and that represents gratifying progress. The problem is that no one can live with deprivation forever, so at some point, every dieter goes off the reservation and starts eating again. The long-term consequences of this type of calorie deprivation are a slower metabolism and less lean muscle mass. Those repercussions make it more difficult to maintain a healthy weight. Not good. Yet, many people repeat this cycle many times. Some even get desperate and succumb to downing Dr. Oz's latest miracle fat-burning pill. The likely result: your wallet is lighter, but the scale doesn't budge.

Get real. It's time to live in the real world, with all of its temptations. Inexpensive, highly processed, calorically dense, extremely tempting food is everywhere. Order a restaurant entrée, and you get two to three servings. Go to McDonald's, and you'll be super-sized. Walk into a Hometown Buffet, and you'll eat until you're about to explode. Walk through the office kitchen, and you'll be lucky to get by scarfing down only a single donut.

Want to lose weight for good? Follow these eight simple practices:

#1: Practice Self-Compassion
Stop hating yourself for being overweight. All the external cues point to overeating. There is nothing wrong with you if you yield to those temptations. But if you want to maintain a healthy weight, you need to plan to be healthy, start from a place of self-compassion, and slowly develop some healthier habits.

#2: Exercise Portion Control
Most overweight people eat too much food. Acquaint yourself with portion sizes, and eat accordingly. Every time you eat out, ask for a takeout box as soon as your entrée arrives. Divide your meal in half, and eat the second serving the next day.

#3: Eat More Fruits and Vegetables
Fruits and vegetables contain lots of healthy nutrients, are low in calories, and fill up your plate. Ditch packaged foods and eat real food. Sub out mega quantities of starches for healthier alternatives.

#4: Get Adequate Sleep
Research shows that scrimping on sleep leads to weight gain. Your hunger signals do not have time to properly reset. Plus, you'll likely mistake your tiredness for hunger and eat more than you should.

#5: Drink Water
Drink a minimum of eight glasses of fluid per day — and more when you exercise. Coffee, tea, and soup all count. Keeping hydrated will aid in digestion and keep you feeling a little full. You won't make the mistake of thinking you're hungry when you're really thirsty.

#6: Eat Breakfast
Your mother was right. People who've lost significant amounts of weight and kept it off for years share the common practice of

eating breakfast. Consider the fact that your body has been fasting while you were sleeping. If you expect your body and brain to get in gear, they need fuel. A cup of joe and a croissant won't do. Aim for a meal that includes protein and complex carbohydrates.

#7: Be a Little Bad
As a Wellness Coach, I counsel my clients to "be a little bad." The point is to develop healthy, sustainable habits. Resist the temptation to go into diet mode. Continue to indulge in your favorite foods so you don't crave them and overdo it when your resolve wears thin. Just enjoy them in moderation. Deprivation is no way to live.

#8: Exercise Regularly
While exercise will not burn enough calories to help you lose a lot of weight, it's an absolute necessity for maintaining a healthy weight. Exercise also keeps many diseases at bay, including Alzheimer's disease. Plus, you'll find that when you start paying attention to your body and moving it more, you're more likely to make healthy food choices as well.

As much as we try to tell ourselves differently, deep down, we realize that quick fixes don't work in the long run. Why not give these simple tips a try and start adopting healthier habits?

SIX DIET AND NUTRITION MYTHS DEBUNKED

Are you confused about what you should and shouldn't be eating? Are eggs good for you, or will they give you a heart attack? Have you been enjoying your nightly glass of red wine only to read the latest study, which claims that *any* amount of alcohol is bad for your health? Tired of being whipsawed? Here's the lowdown on six prominent myths about diet and nutrition:

Myth #1: Diets Work

Many dieters are successful in the short term and are motivated by the fact that the weight comes off fast. The problem is that eventually all dieters get tired of deprivation and go back to their old habits. The only answer is to learn how to live in the real world with all of its fast-food temptations.

Myth #2: You Can Exercise the Weight Off

Tempted to join a gym and maybe even hire a personal trainer to get the weight off? Don't. We overestimate how many calories are burned by exercise. Just one example proves my point: go for a moderate jog for forty-five minutes, and you get to eat eight Oreos. Woo-hoo! Maintaining a healthy weight is largely a function of what you put in your mouth. Exercise is an important ingredient of a healthy life, but it is not an effective weight-loss technique.

Myth #3: Skipping Breakfast Saves Calories

Do you skip breakfast because you 1. are too busy to eat, 2. don't feel hungry, or 3. think you'll save calories by not eating until lunchtime? If so, you're likely to be overweight. Think about it. Your body has been fasting while you were sleeping, and now you expect it to get up and go mentally and physically with no fuel. Would you expect your car to run without gas? Many studies demonstrate that skipping breakfast only results in back-loading extra calories late in the day and making poor food choices.

Myth #4: Dr. Oz Has All the Answers

Dr. Oz has marketed himself as the nutrition guru of America. Every week he uses his wide-reaching media outlets to get his audience all excited about a magic pill that will melt the excess weight right off your body. Have you tried raspberry ketones, garcinia cambogia, or green coffee beans? I bet the only thing that got lighter was your wallet. Think about it: he trumpets a new product every week. Doesn't that make you wonder about last week's "miracle?"

Myth #5: Your Body Needs a Colon Cleanse

Colon cleanses involve extreme calorie deprivation. As a result, you will likely lose weight immediately. However, no one can live on juice alone for long. Many people who go this route seem to be doing some sick kind of penance to punish themselves for their bad eating habits. The body is a self-cleaning machine. Enough said.

Myth #6: There Are "Magic Foods"

Blueberries, acai berries, quinoa, kale. Are you tired of them? I am. They all have excellent nutritional value, but so do a lot of other foods. There are no special foods that will make up for eating junk food. Eat real food. Leave the packages on the grocery store shelves, and aim for variety and color on your plate.

Now that the quick fixes are gone, get real. Get healthy.

WHY WE KEEP DOING SOMETHING WITH A 95 PERCENT FAILURE RATE

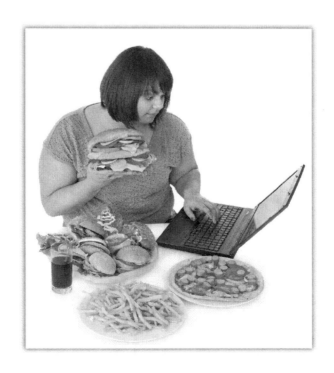

I'm referring to dieting. Any diet. Despite the fact that the vast majority of dieters are doomed to regain not only the pounds they've shed, but to pack on a few more for good measure, we continue to try and try again. At any given time, 108 million Americans are depriving themselves. The typical calorie counter goes on a diet four to five times every year, supporting a $61 billion a year weight-loss industry.

We go gluten-free. We imitate cavemen. We subsist on a few cookies per day. We buy the Magic Bullet so we can eat baby food. And the weight-loss schemes just keep on coming, much like the wind-whipped California wildfires in the third year of a drought.

You don't have to be Albert Einstein to realize that doing the same thing over and over again and expecting different results exemplifies insanity. I coach many long-time yo-yo dieters in my work as a wellness coach, and I have been trying to figure out why so many of us are serial dieters. How do we convince ourselves that the seventeenth diet will succeed even though the first sixteen did not? Here's my take on why diets are so seductive:

#1: **We Experience Instant Gratification:** Dieters lose weight fast, which makes them feel successful. Calorie deprivation will do that for you. The pounds melt off, and suddenly, stepping on your bathroom scale becomes less traumatic.

#2: **We Gain the Illusion of Control:** Diets take real-life temptations out of the equation and make us believe that we are now in control of our eating habits, even if that means eating tasteless packaged food with unpronounceable ingredients or hold-your-nose blended kale drinks.

#3: **We Get to Punish Ourselves:** We know we've been bad, and depriving ourselves feels good because we deserve it. Dieters are punished for their transgressions, much like Catholics going to confession and saying penance. That's why the colon cleanse is so popular.

#4: There's Always a New Flavor of the Month: Strange new diets emerge every year. That's why diet books are perennial best sellers. Just when we think we've tried everything, some enterprising diet guru comes up with another brilliant idea. We convince ourselves that this one is the Holy Grail, and we go for it.

#5: We Believe It's Our Fault That We Failed: We blame our past weight-loss failures not on the diets, but on ourselves. If only we had stuck to the program, we wouldn't have weakened and succumbed to pints of Häagen-Dazs and large bags of Doritos. If we had just had more willpower, we wouldn't be back in our "fat clothes" now.

It's time to realize that no diet is ever going to work in the long run. At some point you'll tire of being crabby and perpetually hungry and return to the very habits that got you in trouble in the first place. The only answer is to learn how to slowly change those habits so that you can live in the real world with its overabundance of tempting, inexpensive, highly caloric food. Habit change is a slow process, but it is the only way to lose weight and maintain a healthy weight for the rest of your life.

So, get real. Get healthy.

MID-FEBRUARY MIGHT BE A GOOD TIME FOR THAT NEW YEAR'S RESOLUTION

I've often wondered why so many people persist in making doomed-to-fail New Year's resolutions year after year. Their likelihood of success: 8 percent. The most popular resolution: lose weight.

I've never made a New Year's resolution in my life. The magic of changing my behavior starting with a new calendar year has always eluded me. Maybe my refusal to join in this annual ritual is grounded in my attitude of not running with the herd. If I wanted to join a gym, why would I choose the most crowded six weeks to make my foray into the sweat brigade? If I wanted to lose twenty pounds, why would I try to do so right after the holiday chocolates had affixed themselves to my backside? If I wanted to get organized (the second most popular resolution for 2014), why would I undertake the task when my house is littered with wrapping debris and pine needles and suffering the effects of being ransacked by toddlers?

No wonder so many people fail. Perhaps many set unattainable goals, like deciding they can miraculously shed twenty-five pounds in two weeks. But the bigger mistake, the one that inevitably condemns the well-intentioned changes to failure, is the fact that they choose January 1 as D day.

Think about it. How do you typically feel on the first day of the new year? Aggravated from several days of having to be nice to relatives who you'd never speak to again but for the familial bond? Exhausted from smiling and making cocktail-party small talk, while stuffing yourself with an endless variety of sweets and fried goodies and holding your stomach in so you don't bust a seam in your holiday finest? Cranky and sleep deprived from too many days of squeezing too much into too few hours? Hungover and bleary-eyed from ringing in the new year? Get my point?

Here's my advice. If you want to change your lifestyle, do it when you have a fighting chance—when you're feeling at least somewhat well rested and when your stress level is manageable. Perhaps mid-February, after the New Year's resolution attempts have already failed, would be a good time.

LOSE THAT DEPRESSION MENTALITY TO STAY HEALTHY

Does the phrase "waste not, want not" ring a bell? Did your mother enroll you in the clean plate club? Then, like me, your parents engrained depression-era mentality in you at an impressionable young age. It's not an easy thing to lose.

I bet you still squeeze every last drop out of the toothpaste tube, add water to the shampoo remnants, and risk life and limb to pick up that lost penny in the middle of the street. This is a commendable, frugal, conservative mind-set. But before you start patting yourself on the back for being a steward of the environment and berating the younger generation for being wasteful, a word of warning is in order.

This otherwise admirable trait may be hazardous to your health when it comes to food. If you still behave as if food can never go to waste because the bread lines are coming back any day, I guarantee you'll join the obesity ranks. I know it sounds alarmist and that it's difficult to dislodge the sentimental memory of a time when the family breadwinner was justifiably proud that he or she was able to put sufficient food on the table. But we now live in a world of superabundance. Face it: the time-honored ritual of delivering milk and eggs to your next-door neighbor before leaving for vacation is now obsolete.

Today, food is everywhere. And it's cheap. Advertisers bombard us with come-ons to wolf down their mouth-watering science projects disguised as food. To make matters worse, the portion sizes are obscene. We buy our sugar and fat-laden food from fast-food drive-thrus or in packages with ingredient lists as long as Sav-On Pharmacy registers receipts. Warehouse stores like Costco and Sam's Club have conditioned us to buy ginormous bags of kettle chips by offering this oversize quantity at a 60 percent discount. "Betcha can't eat just one." And everyone knows you can't munch on chips without ranch dressing, and that comes in a sixty-four-ounce jug.

Many of us don't cook much anymore. Instead we frequent restaurants and unconsciously devour portion sizes meant for two or three. Or we host a dinner party and cook enough food to feed a Super Bowl team before kickoff, just to make sure no one leaves our table even the slight bit peckish. The result is a refrigerator brimming with leftovers that we feel compelled to finish, lest we let good food go to waste.

We boomers need to change our ways. Here are some new rules to live by:

- Don't let packaged food with polysyllabic ingredients jump into your shopping.

- Become friends with your trash can and garbage disposal.

- Don't buy supersize quantities and tempt overindulgence.

- If you have children, make separate meals for yourself.

- Beg your dinner guests to take leftovers with them.

GET THAT BODY MOVING

Kids never stop moving. Turns out, that's what our bodies prefer. The older we get, the more likely you'll find us sitting at our desks for hours on end or plopped down on the couch. Excessive sitting not only slows down your metabolism, it is actually hazardous to your health. Most of us will never spend one or two hours per day working out. But that doesn't mean you can't be healthy. The answer: exer-snacks — short bursts of movement that let your body know you want it to keep functioning at optimal capacity instead of going into computer save mode.

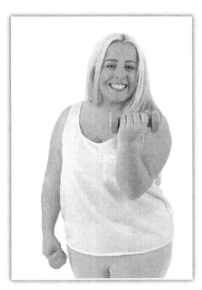

CONFESSIONS OF A FITNESS FANATIC

Health and fitness are my life now at age fifty-nine. Most normal human beings would label me certifiable or a fanatic since I work out with my husband at the crack of dawn every day. And I mean every day. That includes Christmas Day and vacations. When we travel, the adequacy of the workout room determines our choice of hotel. It wasn't always this way.

While many people are active through high school and then slack off, true to form, I followed the opposite path. My all-girls New York City Catholic high school had no gym, so every Friday we changed into our nondescript black leotards and took our smelly feet to the auditorium for yoga. The hippie teacher schooled us in meditation as well, but the nuns never caught on or they surely would have eliminated that pagan practice.

My next foray into regular exercise consisted of an ill-conceived bicycling trip to Quebec City and its surroundings one summer when I was home from Penn State. This was entirely my mother's idea. We prepared for the foolhardy adventure by riding our recently purchased, bottom-of-the-line bikes around the Central Park Reservoir for a total of three or four Saturdays. When we headed out, neither of us had ever changed a tire nor ridden a bicycle with all our worldly belongings in carefully balanced saddlebags over the rear tire. Her harebrained plan called for our two-wheelers to be our sole means of transportation, with overnight respites in cheap roadside motels. The trip began inauspiciously when I managed to get a flat just outside the Quebec Airport terminal. Then, much to my mom's consternation, a few days into this two-week escapade, I came down with a fever, undoubtedly brought on by her insistence that we pedal nonstop during a two-day driving rainstorm. And that wasn't even the worst part. Once on the road, I realized that my mom rode so slowly, she challenged the laws of physics to keep her bicycle upright. So, I spent most of the trip hanging out by the side of the road, killing time, waiting for her to catch up. The end result: I was cured of a desire to exercise for several years to come.

It wasn't until my second year in law school that I contracted the fitness bug. It happened one day when I was camping out at my boyfriend's apartment. I decided I was tired of killing time in the mornings while he ran around the polo fields in Golden Gate Park and returned invigorated with a smile on his face. So, I agreed to give it a try. At first I could barely complete the three-quarter-mile circuit. But I was hooked—not because I fell in love with running or burned up the track with lightning speed, but because I discovered it was the perfect stress antidote. My habitual running is what got me through law school and the California bar exam without a nervous breakdown. Once in law practice, exercise as stress relief saved me from killing my difficult boss and ending up in the slammer.

Through the years, my exercise regimen has changed from running to cycling and now to spin classes, workout machines, and lifting. In deference to my advanced years, I no longer do killer workouts, like the trendy CrossFit, or daredevil sports. As I enter my seventh decade, I've become wary of any new twinge I feel while working out, as I know that even the slightest injury will take months to heal. So, I go with the flow, change it up as my body ages, and just keep moving. It requires effort, and there are certainly days when sleeping in is all too tempting, but it's all about consistency. I know I'm not getting out of this life alive, but I'd like to feel good until that night when I die peacefully in my sleep.

A SUREFIRE WAY TO REV UP YOUR METABOLISM

If you're a boomer, you've probably noticed that suddenly you're lugging around a few extra pounds despite your stepped-up efforts to resist scrumptious desserts and go to the gym. Reaching mid-life and dreading the readout on the bathroom scale go hand in hand. Now that I'm in my sixth decade, it seems that my metabolism has slowed from its childhood hummingbird pace to a sloth-worthy crawl. When I think of all the junk-food calories I was able to scarf down in my youth while maintaining a healthy weight, I momentarily long to be twenty years old again.

If you're like me, your first reaction was denial. You racked your brain, thinking that maybe you'd started a new medication that was responsible for the weight gain. No such luck. Maybe you even visited your doctor, secretly hoping you might have some treatable medical condition, like an underactive thyroid. No dice.

It's time to face reality. Unfortunately, weight gain in your boomer years is mostly likely due to the ravages of "normal aging." Think of your body as a planned obsolescence machine. It's designed to produce offspring and then slowly wind down. That's why kids run around all day while we're content to sit on the couch and watch spectator sports.

What accounts for the slowdown in fat burning as we age? In a word, *sarcopenia*. Never heard of it? Neither has spell check. The word was invented in 1988 by Professor Irwin Rosenberg, MD, director of Tufts University's Human Nutrition Research Center on Aging, to describe the noticeable decline in skeletal muscle mass that occurs as we age. Aging specialists like Dr. Bruno Vellas, president of the International Association of Gerontology and Geriatrics, are predicting that "in the future, sarcopenia will be known as much as osteoporosis is now."

What's the relationship between shrinking muscles and excess pounds? Think of your muscles as your body's fuel burning engine. If you downsize from a V8 to a four-cylinder, your body will use less fuel. That's good for cars but bad for humans. The end result is that as you lose muscle, your body burns fewer calories and the unused fuel gets stored as fat. Before you know it, you have muffin top and can't fit into your jeans.

Beginning at age thirty, we lose, on average, about six pounds of muscle per decade. Between the ages of thirty and eighty, our muscle mass can shrink a whopping 40 to 50 percent. As muscle weakness progresses, it eventually leads to decreased mobility and an increased likelihood of becoming disabled.

So what can you do to combat sarcopenia? The cure comes from the space program, since antigravity produces sarcopenia-like effects in astronauts. Resistance training, or weight lifting, works by putting a load on a muscle, creating small tears, which repair themselves and result in the muscle tissue increasing in size and strength.

And you need not spend hours in the gym. A moderate amount of resistance training done on a regular basis will rev up your engine again. The American College of Sports Medicine recommends twenty to thirty minutes of training, two to three times per week.

Don't try using your advanced age as an excuse not to start rebuilding muscle. A group of wheelchair-bound ninety-year-olds in an assisted living facility showed remarkable improvement after performing thirty minutes of resistance training for fourteen weeks. On average, they added four pounds of lean muscle while eliminating three pounds of fat. They also increased their leg strength by 80 percent and their upper body strength by 40 percent. So get lifting!

MY TOP TEN PEEVES AT THE GYM

If you spend any amount of time in the gym, over time you notice that certain things get mighty annoying. Here is my Top Ten list:

- My personal trainer invents wacko, extremely challenging, and perhaps dangerous workouts that I'll never be able to replicate on my own.

- The only machines without bodies on them have Out of Order signs.

- The staff vacuums around me while I'm trying to work out.

- I go to take a shower only to be barraged by litter-covered floors, hair-clogged drains, colorful mold, dirty towels strewn everywhere, and overflowing toilets.

- The music volume is so loud, even my earbuds can't block it out.

- My fellow gym-goers assume their mothers will come by to remove their used tissues, gums, nutrition-bar wrappers, and caked-on, stinky sweat.

- Arnold Schwarzenegger types make their presence known with loud grunting and forcefully throwing weights on the floor.

- People reserve "their" machines by putting all their junk on them and then go and do other things for a half hour.

- Someone acts as if he or she has his or her own personal treadmill by monopolizing it for two hours while the rest of us cool our heels.

- Your fellow gym-goers use weight-machine benches as chairs, where they park themselves for extended periods of time, chatting with their friends, reading, or staring off into space.

Here are some tips for selecting a gym that you will like in the long run:

- Find a gym that is close to your home or your office so you won't have any excuse to not stop by.

- Check out the class schedule and instructors before you join.

- Visit the gym at the times you intend to use it to see how crowded it is.

- Take a shower in the locker room before you sign up.

- Ask if the gym limits the number of members.

- Ask about past fee increases.

- Do a walk-around and see how many machines are out of order.

- Ask about locker thefts.

- Talk to long-time members to see if they're still happy with the gym.

- Make sure the temperature is to your liking and that you won't be freezing or burning up while working out.

EXER-SNACKS: THE BEST WAY TO GET YOUR BODY MOVING

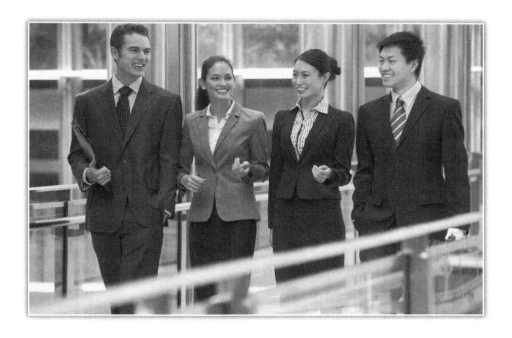

Isn't it ironic that we have so many modern conveniences but can't find the time to take care of ourselves? According to the Centers for Disease Control and Prevention, a whopping 80

percent of US adults don't meet the minimal exercise guidelines—a paltry two-and-a-half hours per week of aerobic exercise and some minimal resistance training twice a week. Not exactly a big-time commitment. We spend more time than that making Starbucks runs, mindlessly watching silly videos, and admiring pet pictures on Facebook.

It's common knowledge that exercise is the magic health pill. It helps with weight maintenance, keeps many diseases at bay, promotes restful sleep, and reduces stress. It even revitalizes your brain health and helps ward off Alzheimer's disease.

So, why don't we take the time to exercise? Has a lethargy plague broken out? No. We just need an attitude adjustment.

Exer-Snacks

Our exercise mind-set is typically a single fixed routine. For example, your habit may be a one-hour visit to the gym. Or maybe you lace up your shoes and hit the road for three miles. Inevitably, stuff happens, and we find ourselves unable to squeeze in our prescribed exercise routine. The result? We do nothing at all. We tell ourselves we'll make it a priority tomorrow.

Attitude adjustment: Studies have found that brief bouts of exercise—as little as ten minutes, rather than a sustained workout of thirty minutes—actually produce superior health benefits, such as controlled blood sugar and hypertension. It may be that we try a little harder with a closer finish line. And most of us find the short stints more enjoyable than the marathon sessions.

Create opportunities for exer-snacks:

- Take a short break and walk around the block.

- Walk to your takeout restaurant to pick up lunch.

- Stand instead of sit during a conference call.

- Talk a walk after you eat dinner.

- Host a walking meeting.

- Walk the airport corridors while waiting for takeoff.

Think Outside the Gym

When we decide it's finally time to get in shape, what do we do? We typically join a gym and maybe even hire a personal trainer. Despite our good intentions, 67 percent of people who have gym memberships never use them. Clearly, forking over an average of fifty-eight dollars per month doesn't do the trick. The truth is, a lot of people hate going to the gym and look for excuses to avoid setting foot in their prepaid health club.

Attitude adjustment: Broaden your horizons about what qualifies as "exercise." The idea is to move your body regularly throughout the day. Lose the idea that the gym is the only place where exercise happens. A killer workout is not the goal. Rather, consistency is the key to staying healthy. There are endless ways to get your body moving. Find things that you like to do. Don't force yourself to walk on the treadmill if it's your version of hell on earth. You won't stick with it for long.

Let Me Count the Ways to Exercise

- Go dancing.

- Dig in the garden.

- Clean your house.

- Take a class at a specialty gym: yoga, Pilates, kickboxing.
- Go for a hike.
- Ride your bicycle.

With exer-snacks and frequent body movement, you will get healthy!

THE DOWNSIDE OF BEING FIT AND LEAN

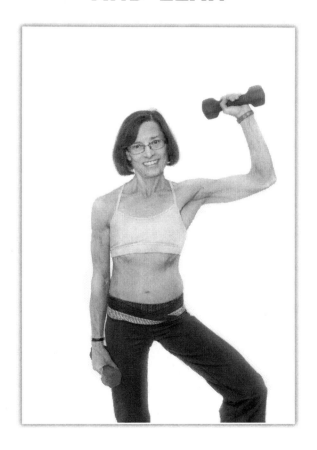

My husband was shopping for a workout outfit for me recently at a fitness store and unsure what size bra top to buy for me. The clerk logically asked him for my bra size. My husband replied, "She doesn't wear a bra." The employee persisted, "Well, what cup size is she?" Somewhat annoyed, my husband then blurted out, "She has no boobs." The flabbergasted woman had no response.

The truth is, I have microscopic boobs. Phil Mickelson's are bigger. Perhaps my husband might have more judiciously said that I'm "fashion-model sized" up top, but I'm OK with his answer. Lucky for me, my husband is a leg and butt man.

For most women, boob size is a big deal, especially in SoCal, where I live. A ridiculously high percentage of women at my health club have suspiciously perky, ginormous breasts. I don't get it. Do they do it to make themselves feel more attractive, or are they out to snag some hard-bodied stud? I hear stories of teenaged girls whose parents buy them boob jobs for their eighteenth birthdays. I find this sad.

For most of my youth, I was a good B cup. I always found bras uncomfortable, but since I was practicing law, I had to endure so as not to have my nipples on display during trial. My body must have sensed my bad attitude because I developed a small cyst due to brassier-to-skin contact, resulting in many additional tests that involved smashing and tugging at what little I had, added doses of radiation, and worry about breast cancer. When I retired from law, I rewarded myself by banishing the nonfunctional undergarment. Miraculously, the offending cyst reabsorbed and never reappeared.

Once I started my career as a personal trainer and wellness coach and had more time to focus on living a healthy life, I gained muscle and lost some flab, much of it from my already marginally sized "girls." Oh well. The only way to be a lean, calorie-incinerating machine and have normal-sized knockers is to go under the surgeon's knife. Not my choice.

I can't say I'm terribly upset to be flat-chested at fifty-nine. It has a lot of advantages. Nothing gets in the way of my golf swing, I don't get whiplash when I run, and gravity and age have not reshaped my boobs into teardrops at my waist. While it's true that most of my sweaters, tops, and dresses look like something has gone missing on top, I don't let that worry me. I'm keeping my fingers crossed that this layering style will stay in vogue until my demise.

TAKE YOUR STRESS DOWN A NOTCH

I spent many years of my life stressed to the max. I was a hard-driving lawyer. Nothing less than perfection was acceptable. I remember literally running up and down the halls when filing deadlines were looming. As a boss, I imposed my impossibly high standards on everyone. At the time, I thought I was setting a good example. Now that I know what chronic stress does to our bodies and brains, I have tried to clean up my act, but it is definitely still a work in progress. Running my own business also ranks high on the stress meter.

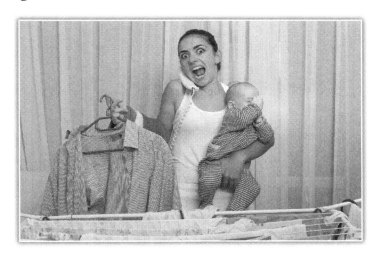

CAN A TYPE A LEARN TO MEDITATE?

I always start my elevator speech by saying, "I'm the world's only type A wellness coach." This is my way of admitting that my personality has failed to adjust along with my career changes. When the United Airlines captain instructs me to "sit back, relax, and enjoy the flight," I haven't a clue how to comply. My husband threw me for a loop one day, in the midst of a discussion about something I was obsessing about, by delivering the news that the point of life is to "be happy." Really? I'd been certain from the time I was still in diapers that the goal was to rack up as many achievements as possible.

Now that I'm a wellness coach, I've been trying to adopt a lifestyle more in line with the Pharrell Williams song "Happy." Because I like to practice what I preach, I've recently delved into the mystical realm of meditation. Unfortunately, my success rate rivals my pathetic attempts to become a passably competent golfer.

To date, I've been a miserable failure at the following:

- Contemplating a raisin for ten minutes

- Slo-mo walking as a way to calm my mind

- Getting through the entry level, ten-minute Headspace app

- *Om*ing my way to peace and solitude

- Refraining from checking my smartphone all the time

During my twenty-three years as a corporate litigator, my workaholic, perfectionist tendencies blossomed like brilliant wildflowers after the spring rains. Not only did I come in earlier and leave later than any other lawyer in the firm, but I also worked almost every weekend and took only one real vacation. My first husband was merely a roommate with benefits. A sleeping brain came only with the aid of Tylenol PM. At age forty-nine, I wisely decided to escape the rat race and explore a new career more compatible with having a life.

After stumbling through several "second" careers, I found my calling and opened my wellness coaching business. For a long time, I'd held out some vain hope that I might mellow after I left the pressure of law practice. Or, as an upside of aging, perhaps a blanket of calm would settle over me like a fog bank on the Golden Gate Bridge. Neither has happened. While I've moved the needle a little toward "Happy," to say I've abandoned my hard-driving ways is like claiming that Betty White has slowed down in her old age.

I buy into the well-documented research that demonstrates the multitude of benefits conferred by sedate brain waves. If the likes of Rupert Murdoch, Bill Ford, Arianna Huffington, Oprah, and Steve Jobs have it nailed, why can't I get it down? Hopefully I'll get there some day. But after a year of trying to instill calm in my gray matter, it's still behaving like a racehorse at the starting gate. That's not to say I haven't made some progress:

So, here are my embarrassingly lame accomplishments to date:

- I now take several vacations per year, if only to keep my husband happy.

- I've learned to lighten up on myself for not equaling my law salary in my new career.

- I've honed my ability to focus on a single task with full attention.

- I'm able to do a Lorie version of mindfulness by focusing only on how my body feels while taking my mid-day walks.

- I start each day by sitting quietly for a minute or two (no more than that) and concentrating on the aroma of a scented candle.

I'm trying to take my own advice to heart. Baby steps are the path to lasting behavior change. I may just learn to walk in a few years.

THREE TIPS FOR STRESSED-OUT PROFESSIONALS

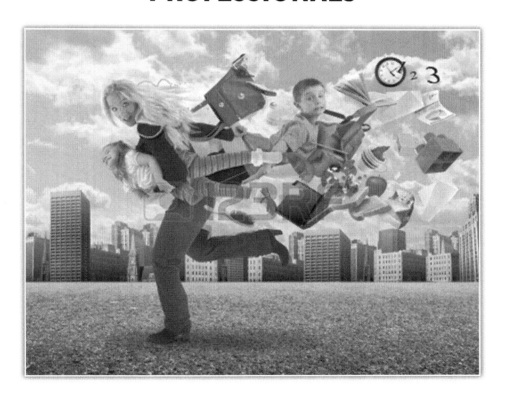

Many of us have very stressful careers. Who hasn't awakened in the middle of the night in a worried panic? Putting in long hours at our jobs is the norm. Many of us end up neglecting our health as a result. Who has time to go to the gym or prepare healthy meals?

But with just a little effort and planning, you can get back on the road to good health habits and feeling better about yourself. Here are some quick tips to help get you there:

1. Plan for Healthy Eating

All it takes to eat healthier during your nonstop workday is a little planning. Bring some healthy snacks to the office. Here are some good options:

- Packaged, presliced apples

- Precooked and peeled hard boiled eggs (Costco)

- Sting cheese

- Your favorite fruits, cut up and packaged in snack-bag portions

- Greek yogurt

2. Ten Minutes of Exercise

Recommended exercise is thirty minutes, five times a week. But you don't have to do it all at once. Here's how to squeeze in ten minutes:

- Walk up and down the stairs in your building.

- Choose a lunch venue that is some distance away from your office so you get a walk with your meal.

- Stand up and walk around in your office during long conference calls.

- Host a walking meeting.
- Buy a stand-up desk.

3. De-Stress

Constant stress causes deleterious physiological changes. Don't turn into an adrenaline junkie. Here are some ways to chill:

- Take five minutes to center yourself and plan for the day before you leave the house.
- Put your exercise plans on your smartphone calendar and consider them doctor-avoidance appointments.
- Take a minute out of your day to do or say something nice to a colleague or loved one.
- Keep a gratitude journal.
- Frame your favorite reality check, inspirational message and place it in plain view on your desk.

HOW TO MAINTAIN YOUR SANITY DURING THE HOLIDAYS

The holidays are supposed to be a joyful time of relaxed gatherings of family and friends. But we all know that's in *Leave it to Beaver* land. Our reality is that we are totally stressed out, frazzled, and sleep deprived and have seemingly endless altercations over parking spots or who was next in the checkout line. Camaraderie comes in the form of being flipped the bird by our fellow motorists.

Are we having fun yet? I don't think so. Sometimes I wish I had the ability to hibernate. I'd be good with sleeping through the holiday season and waking up as the new year dawns and life returns to normal. I've come to dread the onslaught of holiday promos and fake cheer, which now starts *before* Halloween. Things are even crazier this year with more and more retailers succumbing to the temptation to jumpstart sales by moving Black Friday to Thanksgiving Day. Can't we even enjoy our turkey in peace?

I could go on. Instead, I decided to be constructive and offer seven tips to help you keep your wits about you during this insane time of year. It always helps to have a strategy when you go into battle!

Holiday Sanity-Preserving Tips

1. **Emulate Nancy Reagan:** "Just say no." You don't have to go to every event.

2. **Cheat:** If you're the host, don't make everything from scratch. Supplement with some healthy prepared or takeout food.

3. **Squelch Your Perfectionist Tendencies:** The point is to have fun, not to put on the most perfect party in the history of the world.

4. **Act Like a Duck:** We don't get to choose our family. If one of your relatives gets under your skin, just let the remark roll off your back and be polite.

5. **Get Your Shut-Eye:** It will help you make better food choices and have the time and energy to exercise.

6. **Keep Your Body Moving:** Sneak in some exercise, even if it's just ten minutes. Walk down the stairs; park a little further away from the store.

7. **Strategize:** Develop a plan before you go to a party so you won't overindulge. Try eating a healthy snack before you go, alternate glasses of water and wine, and survey all the offerings before you choose.

Enjoy the holidays.

ARE YOU TOO BUSY TO GO TO THE RESTROOM?

Your answer to this question is one litmus test of an overstressed, overscheduled life. It's a sad commentary on contemporary life that many people can't seem to find the time to answer nature's call. Some of us studiously avoid fluids so as not to waste valuable time taking bathroom breaks. We "hold it in" while we multitask our way through life, disregarding the risk of bladder and kidney infections. When we do make the time to visit the restroom, three-quarters of us continue to use our smartphones.

The same pattern applies to our eating habits. We often mindlessly overindulge, oblivious to our body's satiety signals. It's so old school to sit down at a table and give our undivided attention to the plate of food in front of us. Add a dollop of stress to our workday, and off we go to the vending machine to grab a poor-quality chocolate bar or a bag of stale chips. Cooking just takes too long. Even nuking in the microwave wastes several minutes. We prefer to order online, park in the takeout only spot, run in, rush home, and gobble it down before it gets cold. Or we inch our way through the fast-food drive-thru, never missing a beat on our smart devices. Sometimes the food doesn't even grace our doorstep. We scarf it down at seventy miles an hour, like a ravished dog, paying little attention to what we are inhaling unless we get unlucky and ketchup lands on our freshly laundered white shirt.

Many, if not most of us, are "running on empty," as the Jackson Browne song goes. Our constant go-go-go mode may be attributable to technology run amuck, the drive to be the perfect parent, or simply the inability to utter the word no when asked to take on yet another task. No matter. The result is the same — we're rushing through life like so many tornado chasers. Is this any way to live?

This constant adrenaline-fueled pace is taking a toll on our health. Is it any surprise that 43 percent of adults suffer adverse effects from stress and that 75 to 90 percent of all doctor's visits are for stress-related ailments?

We all need to slow down and stop rushing headlong through life like we're on a bullet train. Here are some good ways to decrease your stress level:

- Say *ommm*...

- Move your body.

- Take a real vacation to a place with no cell reception.

- Get your muscles kneaded.

- Get your shut-eye.

- Stop relying on drugs like caffeine, tobacco, and prescription meds to make it through the day.

Try these on for size. You just might discover that a less frenetic pace equates to a more enjoyable life. Remember, we only get one chance to get this right. ;-)

SLOW DOWN: GET YOUR STRESS DOWN TO A REASONABLE LEVEL

Are you rushing through life? Do you find yourself constantly multitasking? Is a good day one where you managed to show up at the right time and place for all your work and personal obligations?

If any of these descriptions fits your lifestyle, I urge you to start getting your stress under control before it's too late. I was a stressed-out workaholic corporate attorney for twenty-three years with no life outside of my legal practice. I was a super achiever at the office and a total failure in my personal life. I treated my husband like a convenient roommate.

If you notice some parallels between my story and your life, rest assured, you can change and achieve a happier, more fulfilling life. I did.

Here are some tips to get you there:

#1: Journal Your Stress Level
The first step to getting your stress under control is to figure out what is stressing you out. Spend a week recording your stress levels periodically and the source of the stress. You'll learn a lot.

#2: Turn Off the Tech
Technology is a wonderful tool, but most of us let it rule our lives. Put it in its place! Designate certain times of day to check for messages and stick to the schedule. Looking at your phone constantly wastes time, creates distractions, and allows your job to take over your personal time.

#3: Just Say No
If you're the perennial volunteer, learn how to keep you hand down. Since your time is finite, taking on added responsibilities necessarily means that you sacrifice something else. Think about what's really important to you. Are you giving your spouse and kids the attention they deserve? Just asking…

#4: Make a Relaxation Appointment
We all need to take a break to recharge on a regular basis. Workaholics eventually reach a point of diminishing returns, and overbooked moms get cranky. Schedule downtime events (e.g., a walk outside, mani-pedi, or a massage) in your smartphone and treat them with the sanctity of a doctor's appointment.

#5: Go Drug-Free
If you fuel yourself with coffee all day, reach for a glass of wine (or two) to relax after a tough day, or pop pills to sleep, your stress is out of control. Craft small, achievable goals to steadily work toward going drug-free.

#6: Practice Mindful Living
In order to enjoy life (isn't that what we're here for?), we need to actually pay attention to it. Research demonstrates that our brains are not capable of multitasking. Focus on a single activity and fully experience it. If you find yourself overeating, try putting your device away and concentrating on your meal. You'll find that the food tastes better, you enjoy it instead of inhaling it, and that you stop eating before you feel stuffed.

#7: Exercise, Exercise, Exercise
One smart thing I did when I was working twelve-hour days was exercise to relieve the day's stress. It really works and offers a host of other health benefits too. Exercise truly is the magic pill.

Reducing stress will also keep your out of the ER. Ninety percent of patients who show up there are being treated for stress-related ailments.

LORIE EBER'S BIO

Lorie Eber earned her Juris Doctor from the University of California, Hastings College of the Law in 1981 and worked in private practice as a corporate litigator for twenty-three years. In 2004, she "retired" and decided to make gerontology (the study of aging) her new career. She has been teaching gerontology online at Coastline Community College since 2006.

After becoming a nationally recognized keynote speaker and a well-known blogger on boomer issues, Ms. Eber decided to pursue a career in health and wellness, which had always been her avocation. She is certified as a personal trainer by the National Academy of Sports Medicine. But since working out is only part of a healthy life, Ms. Eber added to her credentials by studying to become a wellness coach who addresses the three prongs of healthy living: reducing stress, moving your body more, and eating real food in reasonable quantities. She was trained by the Wellcoaches School of Coaching and is also certified by the Mayo Clinic as a Wellness Coach.

Lorie also "walks the walk" on health and fitness. You'll find her working out at the gym with her husband seven days a week at 5:00 a.m. She follows the Mediterranean diet, which provides a balanced diet without deprivation. Ms. Eber has also delved into mindfulness and even attempted to learn how to calm her mind with meditation. The latter is a work in progress.

Lorie Eber Wellness Coaching provides corporate, group, and one-on-one guidance and support to teach clients the skills they need to live a healthy lifestyle. Read Lorie Eber's First Amazon book, *Aging Beats the Alternative and a Sense of Humor Helps*.

For more information about Lorie, visit her website: www.LorieEberWellnessCoaching.com.

Made in the USA
Lexington, KY
08 April 2015